Quick and Easy Keto Vegetarian Cookbook

Lose Weight and Feel Great with Fast and Easy to Do Ketogenic Vegetarian Recipes

Lidia Wong

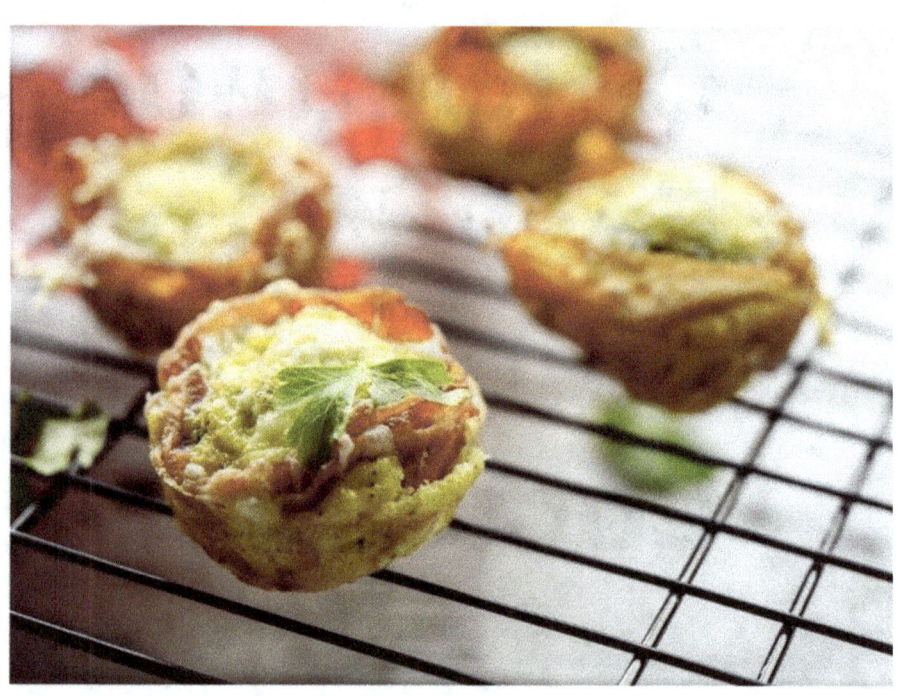

© **Copyright 2021 by Lidia Wong - All rights reserved.**

The content contained within this book may not be reproduced, duplicated or transmitted without direct written permission from the author or the publisher.
Under no circumstances will any blame or legal responsibility be held against the publisher, or author, for any damages, reparation, or monetary loss due to the information contained within this book. Either directly or indirectly.

Legal Notice:
This book is copyright protected. This book is only for personal use. You cannot amend, distribute, sell, use, quote or paraphrase any part, or the content within this book, without the consent of the author or publisher.

Disclaimer Notice:
Please note the information contained within this document is for educational and entertainment purposes only. All effort has been executed to present accurate, up to date, and reliable, complete information. No warranties of any kind are declared or implied. Readers acknowledge that the author is not engaging in the rendering of legal, financial, medical or professional advice. The content within this book has been derived from various sources. Please consult a licensed professional before attempting any techniques outlined in this book.
By reading this document, the reader agrees that under no circumstances is the author responsible for any losses, direct or indirect, which are incurred as a result of the use of information contained within this document, including, but not limited to, — errors, omissions, or inaccuracies.

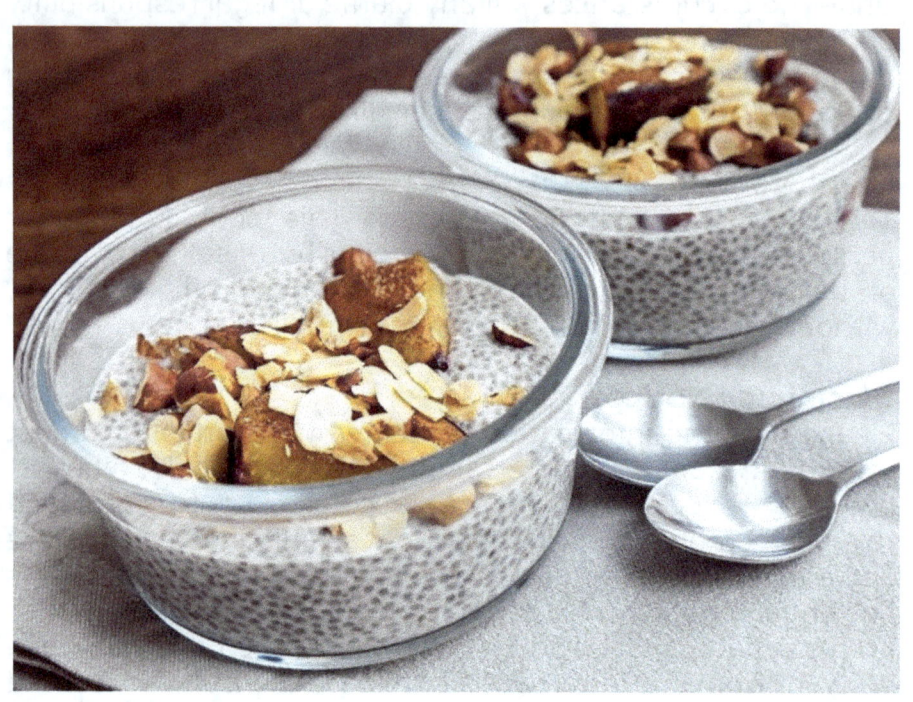

TABLE OF CONTENTS

INTRODUCTION 1

Mint Watermelon Bowl 3

Sweet Cauliflower Rice Casserole 5

Parsley Spread 7

Croque Madame with Pesto 8

Watercress Bowls 11

Egg Salad 12

Gluten Free Asparagus Quiche 14

Yummy Cheese Grits 16

Caprese Casserole 18

Basil Zucchinis and Eggplants 20

Orange Carrots 22

Zucchini Pan 24

Green Beans and Mango Mix 26

Creamy Peas 27

Beans, Carrots and Spinach Side Dish 29

Pilaf 31

Smoky Coleslaw 33

Grilled Artichokes 35

- Carrots and Lime Mix 37
- Garlic Lovers Hummus 39
- Asparagus and Browned Butter 40
- Roasted Radishes 42
- Eggplant Soup 44
- Curried Pumpkin Soup 46
- Two-Potato Soup With Rainbow Chard 48
- Black-Eyed Pea & Sweet Potato Soup 50
- Caramelized Onion And Beet Salad 52
- Savory Seed Crackers 54
- Spinach and Chard Hummus 56
- Red Pepper and Cheese Dip 58
- Cherry shed Coconut Muffins 60
- Zaatar Popcorn 62
- Rice Pizza 63
- Chaffles With Keto Ice Cream 65
- Cauliflower Rice 67
- Queso Blanco Dip 69
- Classic Buttermilk Syrup 71
- Cheese Fries 73
- Lemon Garlic Mushrooms 74
- Cauliflower Asparagus Soup 76

Chard And Sweet Potato Soup 78

Lentils Curry 80

Flax Egg (vegan) 82

Maple-Walnut Oatmeal Cookies 84

Cherry-Vanilla Rice Pudding (Pressure cooker 86

Strawberry Parfaits With Cashew Crème 88

Vegan Chocolate Bars 90

Pina-Colada Cake 92

Chocolate Almond Butter Smoothie 94

Nutmeg Pudding 96

Grapes Vanilla Cream 98

Chocolate Fudge 99

NOTE **101**

INTRODUCTION

The keto diet is the shortened term for ketogenic diet and it is essentially a high-fat and low-carb diet that helps you lose weight, thereby bringing various health benefits. This diet drastically restricts your carb intake while increasing your fat intake; this pushes your body to go into a state know as "*ketosis*". We will tackle ketosis in a bit.

The human body uses glucose from carbs to fuel metabolic pathways—meaning various bodily functions like digestion, breathing, etc.. Essentially, anything that needs energy. Even when you are resting, the body needs fuel or energy for you to continue living. If you think about it, when have you ever stopped breathing, or your heart stopped beating, or your liver stopped from cleansing the body, or your kidneys from filtering blood?

Never, unless you're dead, which is the only time in which the body doesn't need energy. In normal circumstances, glucose is the primary pathway when it comes to sourcing the body's energy.

But the body also has another pathway; it can utilize fats to fuel the various bodily processes. And this is what we call "*ketosis*". And the body can only enter ketosis when there is no glucose available, thus the reason for sticking to a low-carb diet is essential in the keto diet. Since no glucose is available, the body is pushed to use fats—it can either come from the food you consume or from your body's fat reserves—the adipose tissue or from the flabby parts of your body. This is how the keto diet helps you lose weight, by burning up all those stored fats that you have and using it to fuel bodily processes.

That said, if for whatever reason you are a vegetarian, following a ketogenic diet can be extremely difficult. A vegetarian diet is largely free of animal products, which means that food tends to be usually high in carbohydrates. Still, with careful planning, it is possible. This Cookbook will provide you with various easy and delicious dishes to help you stick to your ketogenic diet plan while being a vegetarian.

Enjoy!

Mint Watermelon Bowl

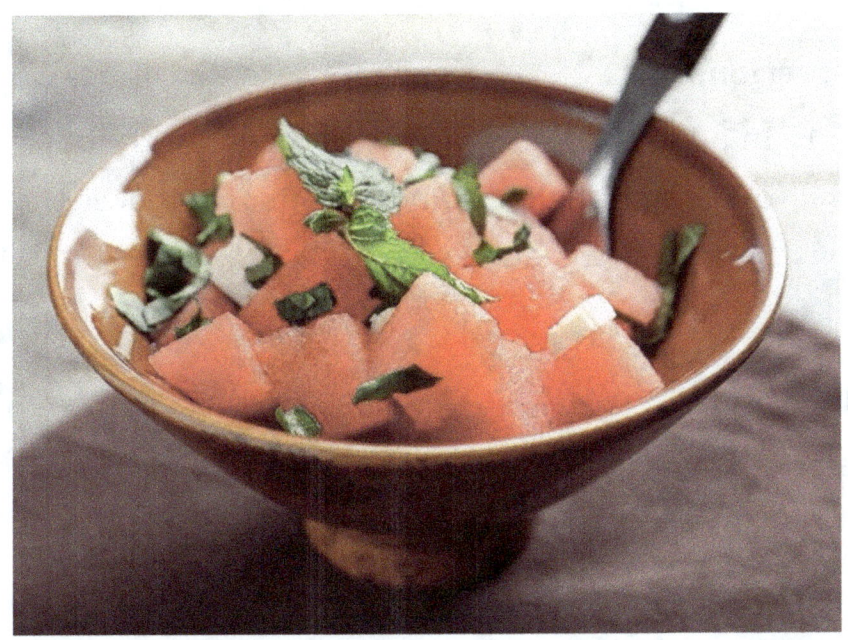

Preparation time: 5 minutes

Cooking time: 0 minutes

Servings: 2

Ingredients:

- 2 cups watermelon, peeled and cubed
- 6 kalamata olives, pitted and sliced
- 1 teaspoon avocado oil

- 1 tablespoon mint, chopped
- ½ tablespoon balsamic vinegar

Directions:

1. In a bowl, combine the watermelon with the olives and the other ingredients, toss, divide into smaller bowls and serve.

Nutrition:

calories 90, fat 3, fiber 1, carbs 7, protein 2

Sweet Cauliflower Rice Casserole

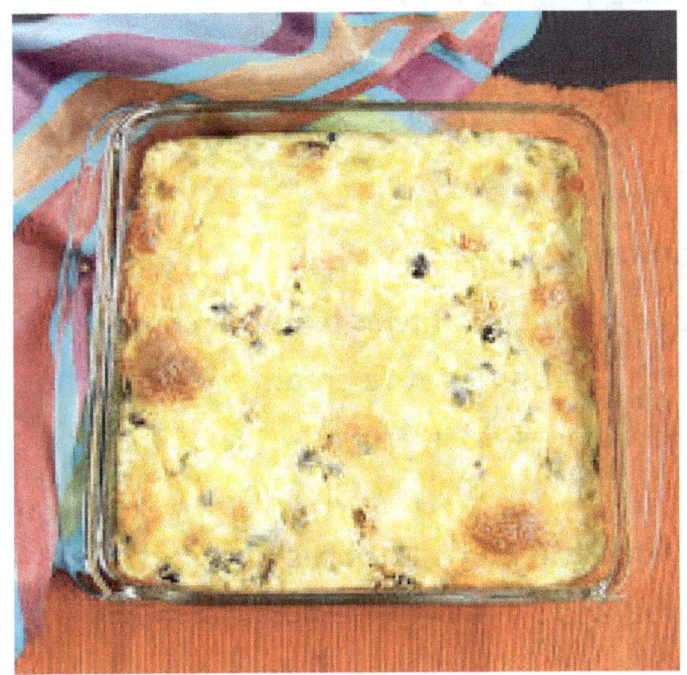

Preparation time: 10 minutes

Cooking time: 1 hour

Servings: 8

Ingredients:

- 1 and ½ cups blackberries
- 1 cup coconut cream
- 1 tablespoon cinnamon powder

- 1 teaspoon ginger, ground
- 2 teaspoons vanilla extract
- 1 cup cauliflower rice
- ¼ cup walnuts, chopped
- 2 cups almond milk

Directions:

1. In a baking dish, combine the cauliflower rice with the berries, the cream and the other ingredients, toss and bake at 350 degrees F for 1 hour.
2. Divide the mix into bowls and serve for breakfast.

Nutrition:

calories 213, fat 4.1, fiber 4, carbs 41, protein 4.5

Parsley Spread

Preparation time: 5 minutes

Cooking time: 0 minutes

Servings: 8

Ingredients:

1. 1 cup parsley leaves
2. 1 cup coconut cream
3. 1 tablespoon sun-dried tomatoes, chopped
4. ¼ cup shallots, chopped
5. 2 tablespoons lime juice
6. 1 teaspoon oregano, dried
7. A pinch of salt and black pepper

Directions:

1. In a blender, combine the parsley with the cream, the tomatoes and the other ingredients, pulse well, divide into bowls and serve for breakfast.

Nutrition:

calories 78, fat 7.2, fiber 1, carbs 3.6, protein 1.1

Croque Madame with Pesto

Preparation Time: 15 minutes

Cooking Time: 30 minutes

Serving: 4

Ingredients:

For the béchamel:

- 2 tbsp unsalted butter
- 1 cup almond milk + extra as needed
- 2 tbsp almond flour
- ½ tsp nutmeg powder
- Salt and black pepper to season
- 4 tbsp grated cheddar cheese

For the pesto:

- ½ cup basil leaves
- ¼ cup grated parmesan cheese
- 1/3 cup toasted pine nuts
- 1 garlic clove, peeled
- ¼ cup olive oil

For the sandwich:

- 1 (7 oz) can sliced mushrooms, drained
- 2 tbsp melted butter

- 4 slices low carb bread
- 3 medium tomatoes, sliced
- 4 slices mozzarella cheese
- 1 tbsp olive oil
- 4 large whole eggs
- Baby arugula for garnishing

Directions:

For the béchamel sauce:

1. Heat the butter and half of the milk in a medium saucepan over medium heat. When the butter melts, whisk in the remaining milk with flour until smooth roux forms.
2. Season with salt, black pepper, and nutmeg. Reduce the heat to low and stir in the cheddar cheese until melted. Turn the heat off and set the sauce aside.

For the pesto:

3. In a food processor, puree the basil, pine nuts, parmesan, garlic, and olive oil.
4. Transfer to a glass jar, cover the lid, and refrigerate until ready to use.

For the sandwich:

5. Preheat the grill to medium-high.
6. Brush both sides of each bread with butter and toast each on both sides until golden.
7. Remove onto a plate and spread the béchamel sauce on one side of each bread, then the pesto, and divide the mushrooms, tomatoes, and mozzarella cheese on top of each bread.
8. One after the other, return each sandwich to the grill and cook until the cheese melts. Transfer to serving plates.
9. Heat the olive oil in a skillet over medium heat and crack an egg into the oil. Cook until the whites are set but the yolks still soft and runny. Place the egg on a sandwich and repeat the same process for the remaining eggs for the rest of the sandwich.
10. Season with salt and black pepper, and garnish with the arugula.
11. Serve warm.

Nutrition:

Calories: 208, Total Fat: 15.3g, Saturated Fat:3 g, Total Carbs: 12 g, Dietary Fiber: 5g, Sugar: 3g, Protein: 8g, Sodium: 73mg

Watercress Bowls

Preparation time: 10 minutes

Cooking time: 0 minutes

Servings: 4

Ingredients:

- 1 cup watercress
- ½ cup cherry tomatoes, halved
- ¼ cup grapes, halved
- 1 tablespoon almonds, chopped
- 1 tablespoon chives, chopped
- ¼ cup baby spinach
- 2 tablespoons avocado oil
- 2 tablespoons lime juice

Directions:

1. In a bowl, combine the watercress with the grapes and the other ingredients, toss well, divide into smaller bowls and serve.

Nutrition:

calories 28, fat 1.8, fiber 1, carbs 2.7, protein 1

Egg Salad

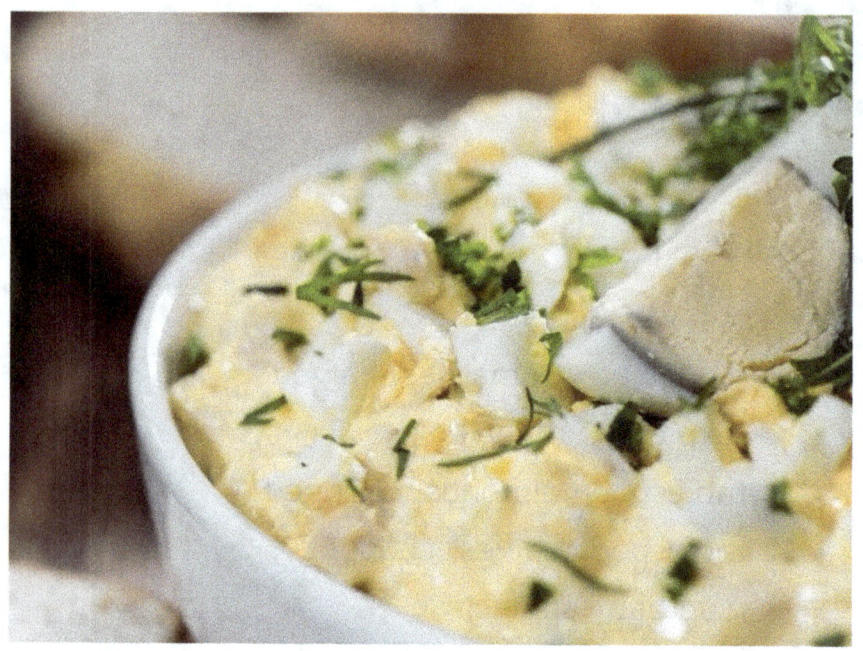

Preparation Time: 15 minutes

Servings: 4

Ingredients:

- 4 eggs, organic, hard-boiled
- ¾ cup celery, diced
- ¼ teaspoon pepper
- 1 teaspoon Dijon mustard

- 1 tablespoon dill, fresh, chopped
- ¼ cup plain yogurt
- ½ teaspoon salt

Directions:

1. Peel your hard-boiled eggs and dice in a large mixing bowl. Add celery, yogurt, dill, pepper, and salt. Mix well. Serve and enjoy!

Nutritional Values (Per Serving):

Calories: 80 Sugar: 1.7 g Fat: 4.7 g Carbohydrates: 2.6 g Cholesterol: 165 mg Protein: 6.8 g

Gluten Free Asparagus Quiche

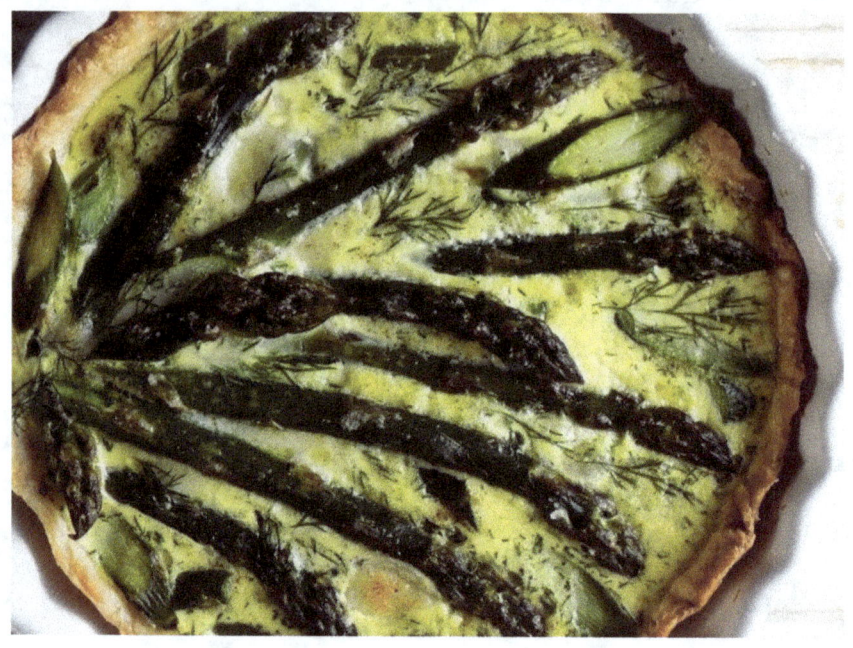

Preparation Time: 1 hour 10 minutes

Servings: 6

Ingredients:
- 5 eggs, beaten
- 1/4 tsp thyme
- 1/4 tsp white pepper
- 1 cup Swiss cheese, shredded
- 1 cup almond milk

- 15 asparagus spears, cut woody ends and cut asparagus in half
- 1/4 tsp salt

Directions:

1. Preheat the oven to 350 °F.
2. Spray a quiche dish with cooking spray and set aside.
3. In a bowl, beat together eggs, thyme, white pepper, almond milk, and salt.
4. Arrange asparagus in prepared quiche dish then pour egg mixture over asparagus.
5. Sprinkle shredded cheese all over asparagus and egg mixture.
6. Place in preheated oven and bake for 60 minutes.
7. Cut quiche into slices and serve.

Nutritional Value (Amount per Serving):

Calories 225 Fat 18 g Carbohydrates 5 g Sugar 3 g Protein 11 g Cholesterol 153 mg

Yummy Cheese Grits

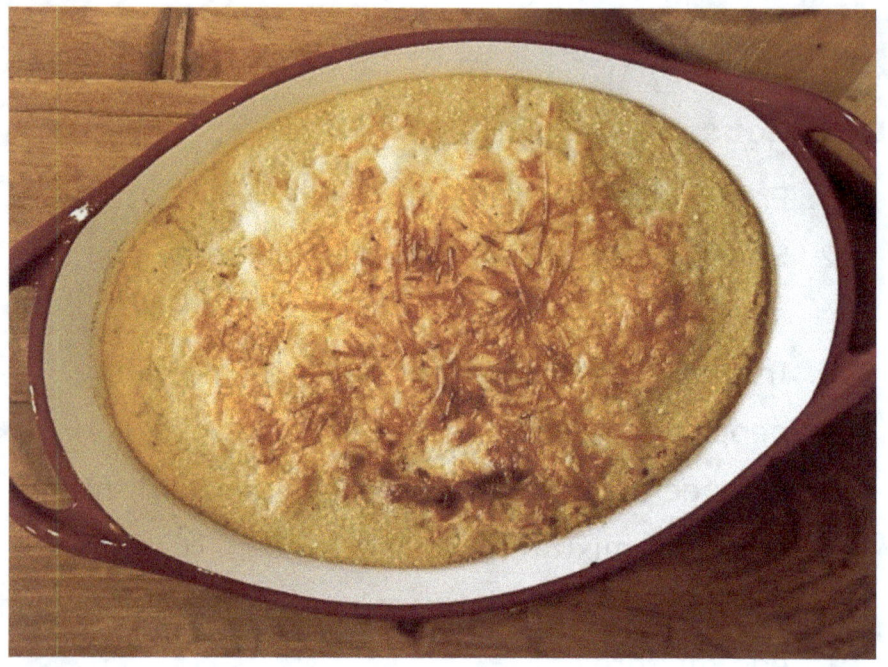

Preparation Time: 10 minutes

Servings: 4

Ingredients:

- 8 large eggs
- 1/2 cup butter
- 1/2 cup cheddar cheese, shredded
- 1/2 cup vegetable broth

- 1 tsp sea salt

Directions:

1. In a bowl, whisk together eggs, salt, and broth.
2. Melt butter in a saucepan over medium heat.
3. Add egg mixture to the saucepan and cook until thickens.
4. Once the mixture is thickened and curds formed then add shredded cheese and stir well to combine.
5. Serve warm and enjoy.

Nutritional Value (Amount per Serving):

Calories 408 Fat 37 g Carbohydrates 1 g Sugar 1 g Protein 17 g Cholesterol 448 mg

Caprese Casserole

Preparation Time: 5minutes

Cooking Time: 20minutes

Serving: 4

Ingredients:

- 1 cup cherry tomatoes, halved
- 1 cup mozzarella cheese, cut into small pieces
- 1 cup vegan mayonnaise
- 2 tbsp basil pesto
- 2 oz. tofu cheese
- Salt and black pepper
- 1 cup arugula
- 4 tbsp olive oil

Directions:

1. Preheat the oven to 350 °F.
2. In a baking dish, mix the cherry tomatoes, mozzarella, basil pesto, mayonnaise, half of the tofu cheese, salt, and black pepper.

3. Level the Ingredients with a spatula and sprinkle the remaining tofu cheese on top.
4. Bake for 20 minutes or until the top of the casserole is golden brown.
5. Remove and allow cooling for a few minutes.
6. Slice and dish into plates, top with some arugula and drizzle with olive oil.
7. Serve.

Nutrition:

Calories:588, Total Fat:59g, Saturated Fat:11g, Total Carbs: 2g, Dietary Fiber:1g, Sugar:1g, Protein:13g, Sodium: 646mg

Basil Zucchinis and Eggplants

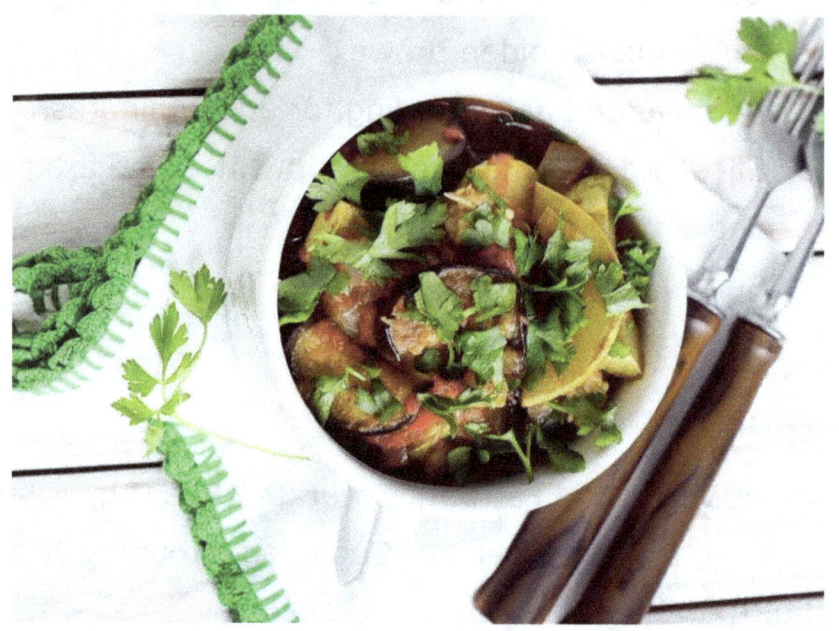

Preparation time: 10 minutes

Cooking time: 20 minutes

Servings: 4

Ingredients:

- 1 eggplant, roughly cubed
- 1 tablespoon olive oil
- 2 zucchinis, sliced

- 2 scallions, chopped
- 1 tablespoon sweet paprika
- 1 teaspoon fennel seeds, crushed
- Juice of 1 lime
- Salt and black pepper to the taste
- 1 tablespoon basil, chopped

Directions:

1. Heat up a pan with the oil over medium heat, add the scallions and fennel seeds and sauté for 5 minutes.
2. Add zucchinis, eggplant and the other ingredients, toss, cook over medium heat for 15 minutes more, divide between plates and serve as a side dish.

Nutrition:

calories 97, fat 4, fiber 2, carbs 6, protein 2

Orange Carrots

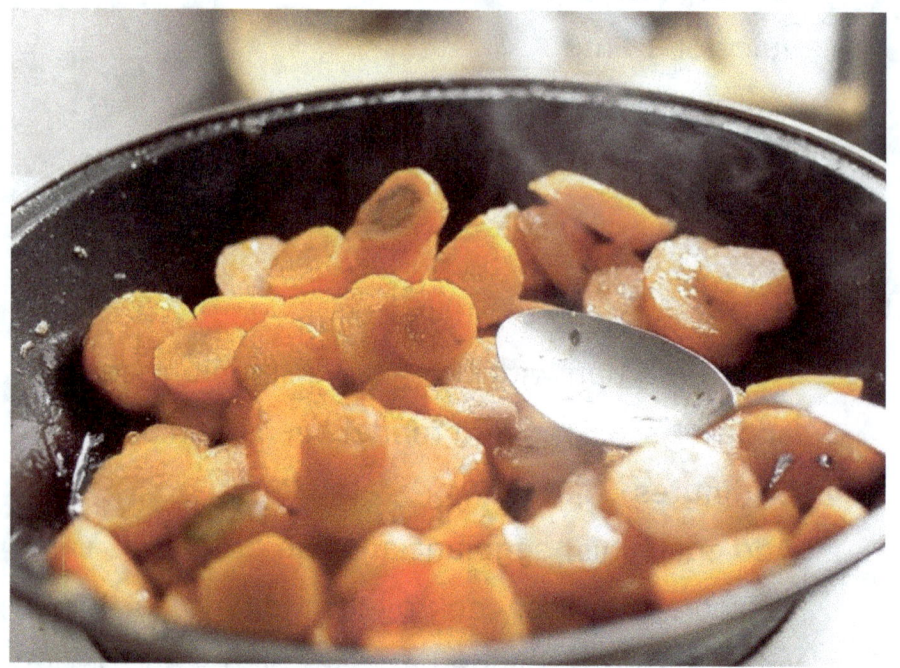

Preparation time: 5 minutes

Cooking time: 25 minutes

Servings: 4

Ingredients:

- 1 pound carrots, peeled and roughly sliced
- 1 yellow onion, chopped
- 1 tablespoon olive oil

- Juice of 1 orange
- Zest of 1 orange, grated
- 1 orange, peeled and cut into segments
- 1 tablespoon rosemary, chopped
- A pinch of salt and black pepper

Directions:

1. Heat up a pan with the oil over medium-high heat, add the onion and sauté for 5 minutes.
2. Add the carrots, the orange zest and the other ingredients, toss, cook over medium heat for 20 minutes more, divide between plates and serve.

Nutrition:

calories 140, fat 3.9, fiber 5, carbs 26.1, protein 2.1

Zucchini Pan

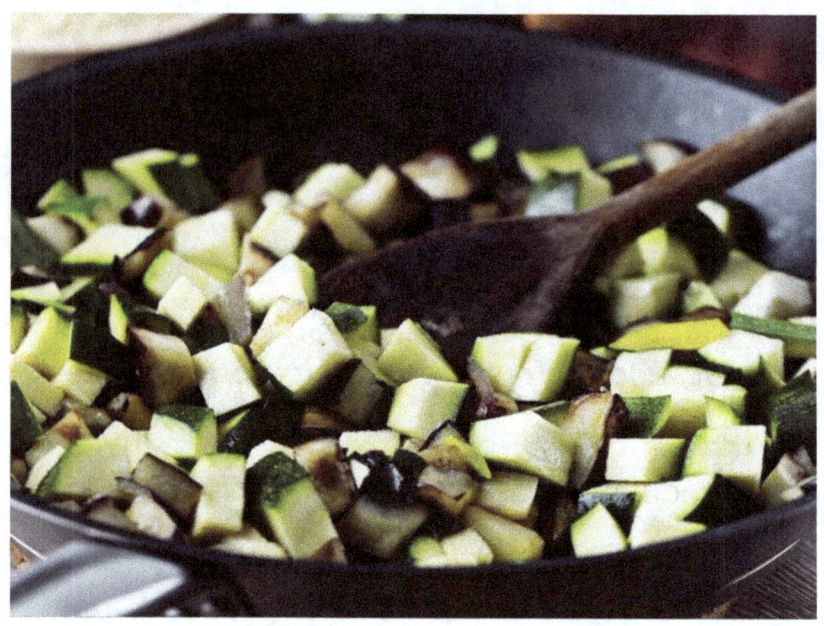

Preparation time: 5 minutes

Cooking time: 20 minutes

Servings: 4

Ingredients:

- 1 pound zucchinis, sliced
- 2 apples, peeled, cored and cubed
- 1 yellow onion, chopped
- 2 tablespoons olive oil

- 1 tomato, cubed
- 1 tablespoon rosemary, chopped
- 1 tablespoon chives, chopped

Directions:

1. Heat up a pan with the oil over medium heat, add the onion and sauté for 5 minutes.
2. Add the zucchinis and the other ingredients, toss, cook over medium heat for 15 minutes more, divide between plates and serve as a side dish.

Nutrition:

calories 170, fat 5, fiber 2, carbs 11, protein 7

Green Beans and Mango Mix

Preparation time: 10 minutes

Cooking time: 20 minutes

Servings: 4

Ingredients:

- 1 pound green beans, trimmed and halved
- 3 scallions, chopped
- 1 mango, peeled and cubed
- ½ cup veggie stock
- 2 tablespoons olive oil
- 1 tablespoon oregano, chopped
- 1 teaspoon sweet paprika
- A pinch of salt and black pepper

Directions:

1. Heat up a pan with the oil over medium heat, add the scallions and sauté for 2 minutes.
2. Add the green beans and the other ingredients, toss, cook over medium heat for 18 minutes more, divide between plates and serve.

Nutrition:

calories 182, fat 4, fiber 5, carbs 6, protein 8

Creamy Peas

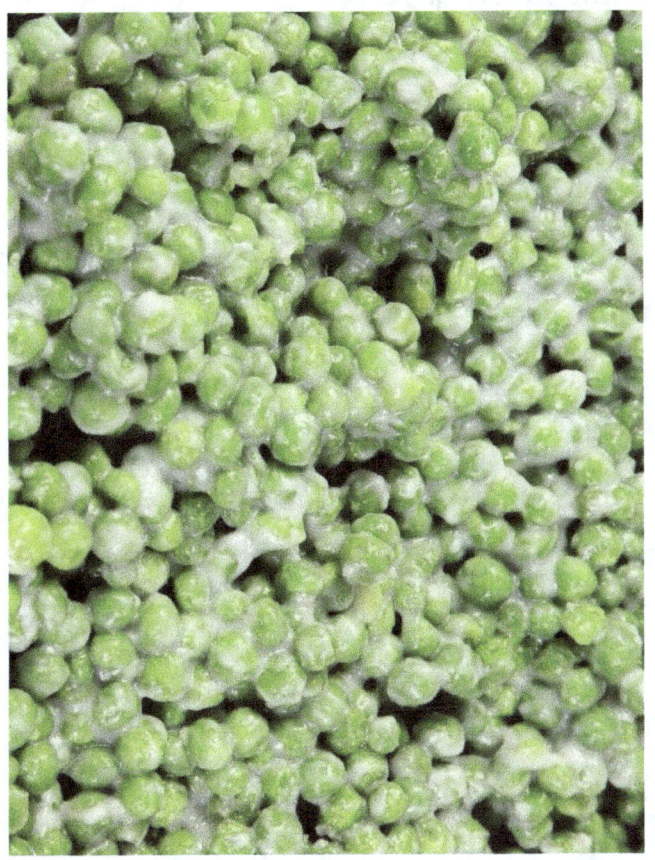

Preparation time: 10 minutes

Cooking time: 20 minutes

Servings: 4

Ingredients:

- 1 cup coconut cream
- 1 tablespoon olive oil
- 1 yellow onion, chopped
- 2 cups green peas
- A pinch of salt and black pepper

Directions:

1. Heat up a pan with the oil over medium heat, add the onion and sauté for 5 minutes.
2. Add the peas and the other ingredients, toss, cook over medium heat for 15 minutes, divide between plates and serve.

Nutrition:

calories 191, fat 5, fiber 4, carbs 11, protein 9

Beans, Carrots and Spinach Side Dish

Preparation time: 10 minutes

Cooking time: 4 hours

Servings: 6

Ingredients:

- 5 carrots, sliced
- 1 and ½ cups great northern beans, dried, soaked overnight and drained
- 2 garlic cloves, minced
- 4 and ½ cups veggie stock
- 1 yellow onion, chopped
- ½ teaspoon oregano, dried
- 5 ounces baby spinach
- 2 teaspoons lemon peel, grated
- Salt and black pepper to the taste
- 3 tablespoons lemon juice
- 1 avocado, pitted, peeled and chopped
- ¾ cup tofu, firm, pressed, drained and crumbled
- ¼ cup pistachios, chopped

Directions:

1. In your slow cooker, mix beans with onion, carrots, garlic, salt, pepper, oregano and veggie stock, stir, cover and cook on High for 4 hours.
2. Drain beans mix, return to your slow cooker and reserve ¼ cup cooking liquid.
3. Add spinach, lemon juice and lemon peel, stir and leave aside for 5 minutes.
4. Transfer beans, carrots and spinach mixture to a bowl, add pistachios, avocado, tofu and reserve cooking liquid, toss, divide between plates and serve as a side dish.
5. Enjoy!

Nutrition:

calories 319, fat 8, fiber 14, carbs 43, protein 17

Pilaf

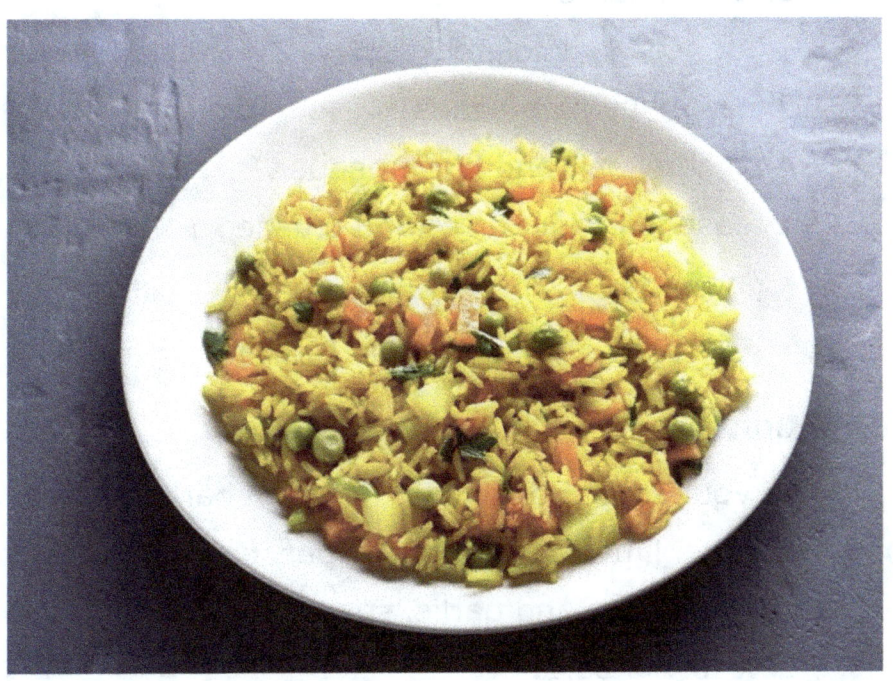

Preparation time: 10 minutes

Cooking time: 7 hours

Servings: 12

Ingredients:
- 2/3 cup wheat berries
- ½ cup wild rice
- ½ cup barley

- 1 red bell pepper, chopped
- 1 yellow onion, chopped
- 1 tablespoon olive oil
- 27 ounces veggie stock
- 2 cups baby lima beans
- A pinch of salt and black pepper
- 1 teaspoon sage, dried and crushed
- 4 garlic cloves, minced

Directions:

1. In your slow cooker, mix rice with barley, wheat berries, lima beans, bell pepper, onion, oil, salt, pepper, sage and garlic, stir, cover and cook on Low for 7 hours.
2. Stir one more time, divide between plates and serve as a side dish.
3. Enjoy!

Nutrition:

calories 168, fat 5, fiber 4, carbs 25, protein 6

Smoky Coleslaw

Preparation time: 10 minutes

cooking time: 0 minutes

servings: 6

Ingredients

- 1 pound shredded cabbage
- 3 tablespoons plain vegan yogurt or plain soymilk
- ⅓ cup vegan mayonnaise
- ¼ cup unseasoned rice vinegar
- 1 tablespoon vegan sugar
- ½ teaspoon salt
- ¼ teaspoon freshly ground black pepper
- ¼ teaspoon smoked paprika
- ¼ teaspoon chipotle powder

Directions

1. Put the shredded cabbage in a large bowl. In a medium bowl, whisk the mayonnaise, vinegar, yogurt, sugar, salt, pepper, paprika, and chipotle powder.

2. Pour over the cabbage, and mix with a spoon or spatula and until the cabbage shreds are coated.
3. Divide the coleslaw evenly among 6 single-serving containers.
4. Seal the lids.

Nutrition:

Calories: 73; Fat: 4g; Protein: 1g; Carbohydrates: 8g; Fiber: 2g; Sugar: 5g; Sodium: 283mg

Grilled Artichokes

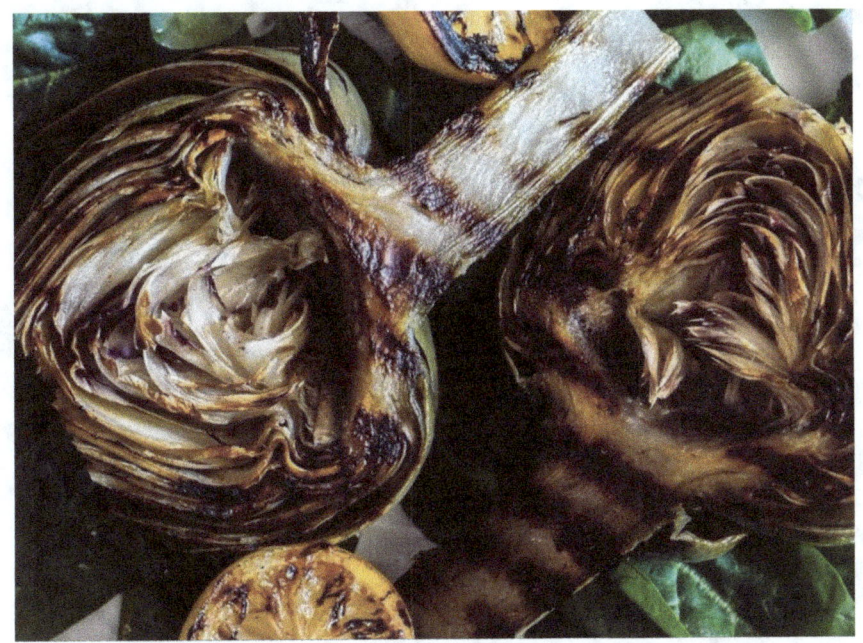

Preparation time: 10 minutes

Cooking time: 25 minutes

Servings: 4

Ingredients:

- 2 artichokes, trimmed and halved
- 1 tablespoons lemon zest grated
- Juice of 1 lemon

- 1 rosemary spring, chopped
- 2 tablespoons olive oil
- A pinch of sea salt
- Black pepper to taste

Directions:

1. Put water in a large saucepan, add a pinch of salt and lemon juice, bring to a boil over medium-high heat, add artichokes, boil for 15 minutes, drain and leave them to cool down.
2. Drizzle olive oil over them, season with black pepper to taste, sprinkle lemon zest and rosemary, stir well and place them under a preheated grill.
3. Broil artichokes over medium-high heat for 5 minutes on each side, divide them between plates and serve.
4. Enjoy!

Nutritional value/serving:

calories 98, fat 7,1, fiber 4,4, carbs 8,5, protein 2,7

Carrots and Lime Mix

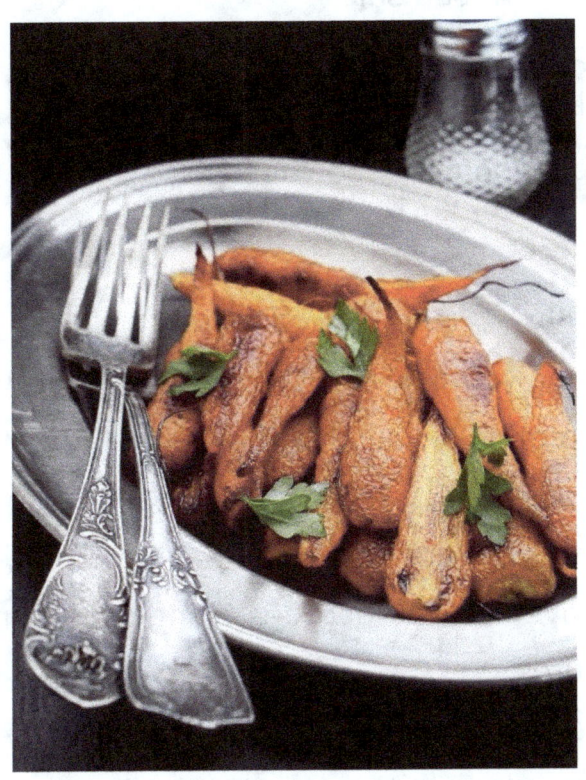

Preparation time: 10 minutes

Cooking time: 30 minutes

Servings: 6

Ingredients:

- 1 and ¼ pounds baby carrots

- 8 garlic cloves, minced
- 3 tablespoons ghee, melted
- A pinch of sea salt
- Black pepper to taste
- Zest of 2 limes, grated
- ½ teaspoon chili powder

Directions:

1. In a bowl, mix baby carrots with ghee, garlic, a pinch of salt, black pepper to taste, chili powder and stir well.
2. Spread carrots on a lined baking sheet, place in the oven at 400 degrees F and roast for 15 minutes.
3. Take carrots out of the oven, shake baking sheet, place in the oven again and roast for 15 minutes more.
4. Divide between plates and serve with lime on top.
5. Enjoy!

Nutritional value/serving:

calories 95, fat 6,6, fiber 2,9, carbs 9,1, protein 0,9

Garlic Lovers Hummus

Preparation Time: 2 mins

Servings: 12

Ingredients:

- 3 tbsps. Freshly squeezed lemon juice
- 15 oz. no-salt-added garbanzo beans
- All-purpose salt-free seasoning
- 3 tbsps. Sesame tahini
- 4 garlic cloves
- 2 tbsps. Olive oil

Directions:

1. Drain garbanzo beans and rinse well.
2. Place all the ingredients in a food processor and pulse until smooth.
3. Serve immediately or cover and refrigerate until serving.

Nutrition:

Calories: 103, Fat:5 g, Carbs:11 g, Protein:4 g, Sugars:2 g, Sodium:88 mg

Asparagus and Browned Butter

Preparation time: 10 minutes

Cooking time: 15 minutes

Servings: 4

Ingredients:

- 5 ounces butter
- 1 tablespoon avocado oil
- 8 tablespoons sour cream
- 1½ pounds asparagus, trimmed
- 1½ tablespoons lemon juice
- A pinch of cayenne pepper
- Salt and ground black pepper, to taste
- 3 ounces Parmesan cheese, grated
- 4 eggs

Directions:

1. Heat up a pan with 2 ounces butter over medium-high heat, add the eggs, some salt and pepper, stir, and scramble them.
2. Transfer the eggs to a blender, add the Parmesan cheese, sour cream, salt, pepper, and

cayenne pepper, and blend everything well.
3. Heat up a pan with the oil over medium-high heat, add the asparagus, salt, and pepper, roast for a few minutes, transfer to a plate, and set aside.
4. Heat up the pan again with the rest of the butter over medium-high heat, stir until brown, take off the heat, add the lemon juice, and stir well.
5. Heat up the butter again, return the asparagus to the pan, toss to coat, heat up well, and divide on plates.
6. Add the blended eggs on top and serve.

Nutrition:

Calories - 160, Fat - 7, Fiber - 2, Carbs - 6, Protein - 10

Roasted Radishes

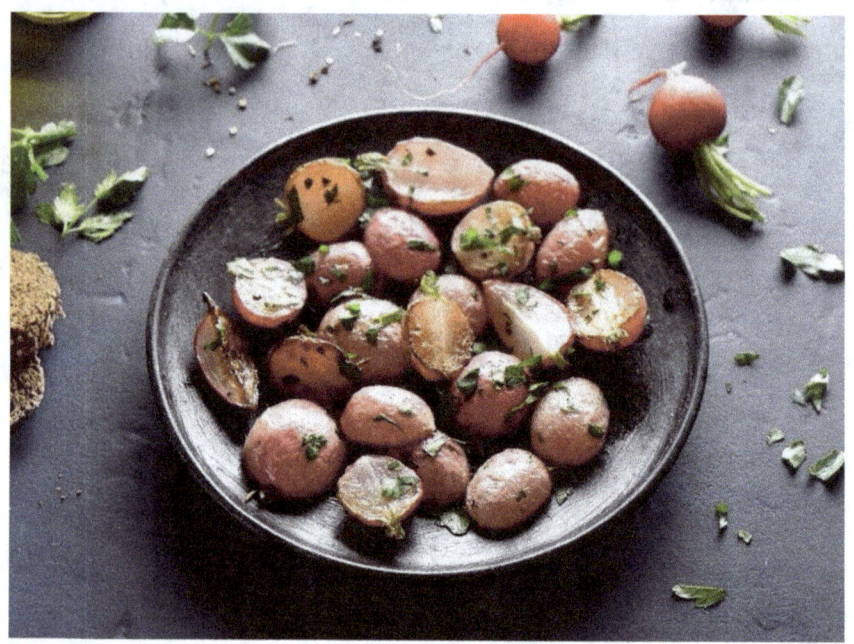

Preparation time: 10 minutes

Cooking time: 35 minutes

Servings: 2

Ingredients:

- 2 cups radishes, cut in quarters
- 2 tablespoons butter, melted
- 1 tablespoon fresh chives, chopped

- Salt and ground black pepper, to taste
- 1 tablespoon lemon zest

Directions:

1. Spread the radishes on a lined baking sheet.
2. Add the salt, pepper, chives, lemon zest, and butter, toss to coat, and bake in the oven at 375 ºF for 35 minutes.
3. Divide on plates and serve.

Nutrition:

Calories - 122, Fat - 12, Fiber - 1, Carbs - 3, Protein - 14

Eggplant Soup

Preparation time: 10 minutes

Cooking time: 50 minutes

Servings: 4

Ingredients:

- 4 tomatoes
- 1 teaspoon garlic, minced
- ¼ onion, peeled and chopped
- 1 bay leaf
- ½ cup heavy cream
- Salt and ground black pepper, to taste
- 2 cups chicken stock
- 2 tablespoons fresh basil, chopped
- 4 tablespoons Parmesan cheese, grated
- 1 tablespoon olive oil
- 1 eggplant, chopped

Directions:

1. Spread the eggplant pieces on a baking sheet, mix with oil, onion, garlic, salt, and pepper, place in an oven at 400 °F, and bake for 15

minutes.
2. Put water in a pot, bring to a boil over medium heat, add the tomatoes, steam them for 1 minute, peel them, and chop.
3. Take the eggplant mixture out of the oven, and transfer to a pot.
4. Add the tomatoes, stock, bay leaf, salt, and pepper, stir, bring to a boil, and simmer for 30 minutes.
5. Add the heavy cream, basil, and Parmesan cheese, stir, ladle into soup bowls, and serve.

Nutrition:

Calories - 180, Fat - 2, Fiber - 3, Carbs - 5, Protein - 10

Curried Pumpkin Soup

Preparation time: 5 minutes

cooking time: 22 minutes

servings: 4 to 6

Ingredients

- 1 tablespoon olive oil
- 1 medium onion, chopped
- 1 (16-ouncecan pumpkin puree or 2 cups cooked fresh pumpkin
- 3 cups vegetable broth, homemade (see Light Vegetable Broth or store-bought, or water)
- 1 garlic clove, minced
- 1 teaspoon grated fresh ginger
- 1 tablespoon hot or mild curry powder
- Salt
- 1 (13.5-ouncecan unsweetened coconut milk
- 1 tablespoon minced fresh parsley, for garnish
- Mango chutney, for garnish (optional)
- Chopped roasted cashews, for garnish (optional)

Directions

1. In a large soup pot, heat the oil over medium heat. Add the onion and garlic and cover and cook until softened, about 7 minutes. Stir in the ginger, curry powder, and cook for 30 seconds over low heat, stirring constantly. Stir in the pumpkin, broth, and salt to taste and bring to a boil. Reduce heat to low, cover, and simmer, uncovered, until the flavors are blended, about 15 minutes.
2. Use an immersion blender to puree the soup in the pot or transfer in batches to a blender or food processor, puree, then return to the pot, and season with salt and pepper to taste. Add coconut milk and heat until hot.
3. Ladle into soup bowls, sprinkle with parsley and a spoonful of chutney sprinkled with chopped cashews, if using, and serve.

Two-Potato Soup With Rainbow Chard

Preparation Time: 5 Minutes

Cooking Time: 45 Minutes

Servings: 6

Ingredients

- 2 tablespoons olive oil
- 1 medium red onion, chopped
- 6 cups vegetable broth, homemade (see Light Vegetable Broth) or store-bought, or water
- 1 medium leek, white part only, well rinsed and chopped
- 2 garlic cloves, minced
- 1 pound red potatoes, unpeeled and cut into 1/2-inch dice
- 1 pound sweet potatoes, peeled and cut into 1/2-inch dice
- 1/4 teaspoon crushed red pepper
- Salt and freshly ground black pepper
- 1 medium bunch rainbow chard, tough stems removed and coarsely chopped

Directions

1. In large soup pot, heat the oil over medium heat. Add the onion, leek, and garlic.
2. Cover and cook until softened, about 5 minutes.
3. Add the broth, potatoes, and crushed red pepper and bring to a boil.
4. Reduce heat to low, season with salt and black pepper to taste, and simmer, uncovered, for 15 minutes.
5. Stir in the chard and cook until the vegetables are tender, about 15 minutes longer and serve.

Black-Eyed Pea & Sweet Potato Soup

Preparation Time: 10 Minutes

Cooking Time: 25 Minutes

Servings: 4

Ingredients

- 1 teaspoon olive oil
- ½ onion, chopped
- 1 garlic clove, minced
- 2 to 3 cups peeled, cubed sweet potato, squash, or pumpkin
- Salt
- 2 cups water
- 1 (15-ounce) can black-eyed peas, drained and rinsed
- 2 tablespoons freshly squeezed lime juice
- 1 teaspoon smoked or regular paprika
- 1 tablespoon sugar
- Pinch red pepper flakes or cayenne pepper
- 3 cups shredded cabbage
- 1 cup corn kernels, thawed if frozen, drained if canned

Directions

1. Heat the olive oil in a large soup pot over medium-high heat.
2. Add the sweet potato, onion, garlic, and a pinch of salt. Sauté for 3 to 4 minutes, until the onion and garlic are softened. Add the water, black-eyed peas, lime juice, sugar, paprika, red pepper flakes, and salt to taste. Bring to a boil and cook for 15 minutes. Add the cabbage and corn to the pot, stirring to combine, and cook for 5 minutes more, or until the sweet potato is tender.
3. Turn off the heat, let cool for a few minutes, and serve.
4. Leftovers will keep in an airtight container for up to 1 week in the refrigerator or up to 1 month in the freezer.

Per Serving (2 cups)

Calories: 224; Protein: 9g; Total fat: 2g; Saturated fat: 0g; Carbohydrates: 46g; Fiber: 10g

Caramelized Onion And Beet Salad

Preparation time: 10 minutes

cooking time: 40 minutes

servings: 4

Ingredients

- 3 medium golden beets
- 2 cups sliced sweet or Vidalia onions
- 1 teaspoon extra-virgin olive oil or no-beef broth
- ¼ to ½ teaspoon salt, to taste
- Pinch baking soda
- 2 tablespoons unseasoned rice vinegar, white wine vinegar, or balsamic vinegar

Directions

1. Cut the greens off the beets, and scrub the beets.
2. In a large pot, place a steamer basket and fill the pot with 2 inches of water.
3. Add the beets, bring to a boil, then reduce the heat to medium, cover, and steam for about 35 minutes, until you can easily pierce the middle

of the beets with a knife.
4. Meanwhile, in a large, dry skillet over medium heat, sauté the onions for 5 minutes, stirring frequently.
5. Add the olive oil and baking soda, and continuing cooking for 5 more minutes, stirring frequently. Stir in the salt to taste before removing from the heat. Transfer to a large bowl and set aside.
6. When the beets have cooked through, drain and cool until easy to handle. Rub the beets in a paper towel to easily remove the skins. Cut into wedges, and transfer to the bowl with the onions. Drizzle the vinegar over everything and toss well.
7. Divide the beets evenly among 4 wide-mouth jars or storage containers. Let cool before sealing the lids.

Nutrition:

Calories: 104; Fat: 2g; Protein: 3g; Carbohydrates: 20g; Fiber: 4g; Sugar: 14g; Sodium: 303mg

Savory Seed Crackers

Preparation time: 5 minutes

cooking time: 50 minutes

servings: 20 crackers

Ingredients

- ¾ cup pumpkin seeds (pepitas
- ½ cup sunflower seeds
- ½ cup sesame seeds
- 1 teaspoon minced garlic (about 1 clove)
- 1 teaspoon tamari or soy sauce
- ¼ cup chia seeds
- 1 teaspoon vegan Worcestershire sauce
- ½ teaspoon ground cayenne pepper
- ½ teaspoon dried oregano
- ½ cup water

Directions

1. Preheat the oven to 325 ºF.
2. Line a rimmed baking sheet with parchment paper.
3. In a large bowl, combine the pumpkin seeds,

sunflower seeds, sesame seeds, chia seeds, garlic, tamari, Worcestershire sauce, cayenne, oregano, and water.
4. Transfer to the prepared baking sheet, spreading out to all sides.
5. Bake for 25 minutes. Remove the pan from the oven, and flip the seed "dough" over so the wet side is up. Bake for another 20 to 25 minutes, until the sides are browned.
6. Cool completely before breaking up into 20 pieces. Divide evenly among 4 glass jars and close tightly with lids.

Nutrition (5 crackers):

Calories: 339; Fat: 29g; Protein: 14g; Carbohydrates: 17g; Fiber: 8g; Sugar: 1g; Sodium: 96mg

Spinach and Chard Hummus

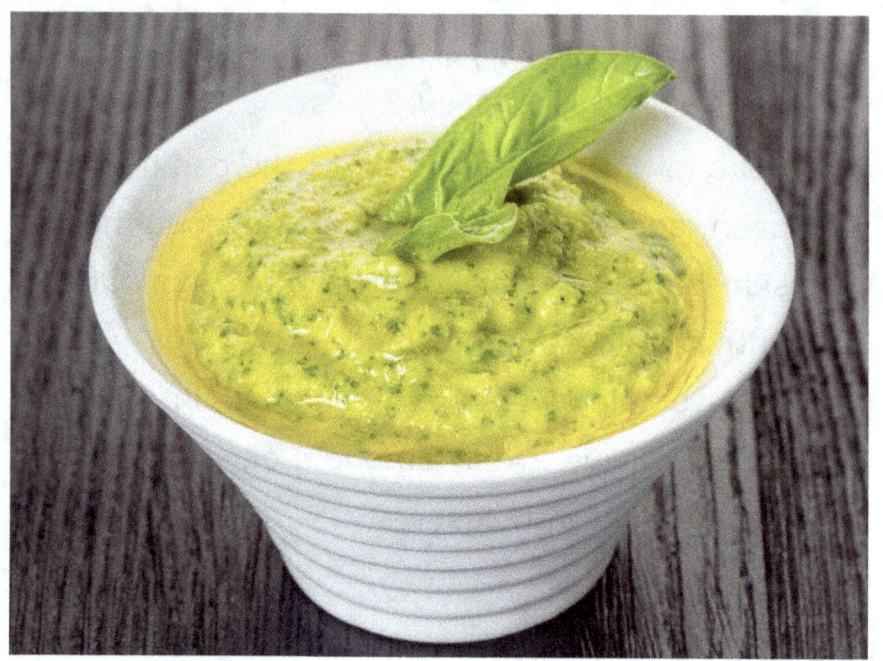

Preparation time: 10 minutes

Cooking time: 10 minutes

Servings: 4

Ingredients:

- 2 cups baby spinach
- 2 garlic cloves, minced
- 2 cup chard leaves

- 2 tablespoons olive oil
- ½ cup coconut cream
- ¼ cup sesame paste
- A pinch of salt and black pepper
- Juice of ½ lemon

Directions:

1. Put the cream in a pan, heat it up over medium heat, add the chard, garlic and the other ingredients, stir, cook for 10 minutes, blend using an immersion blender, divide into bowls and serve.

Nutrition:

calories 172, fat 4, fiber 3, carbs 7, protein 8

Red Pepper and Cheese Dip

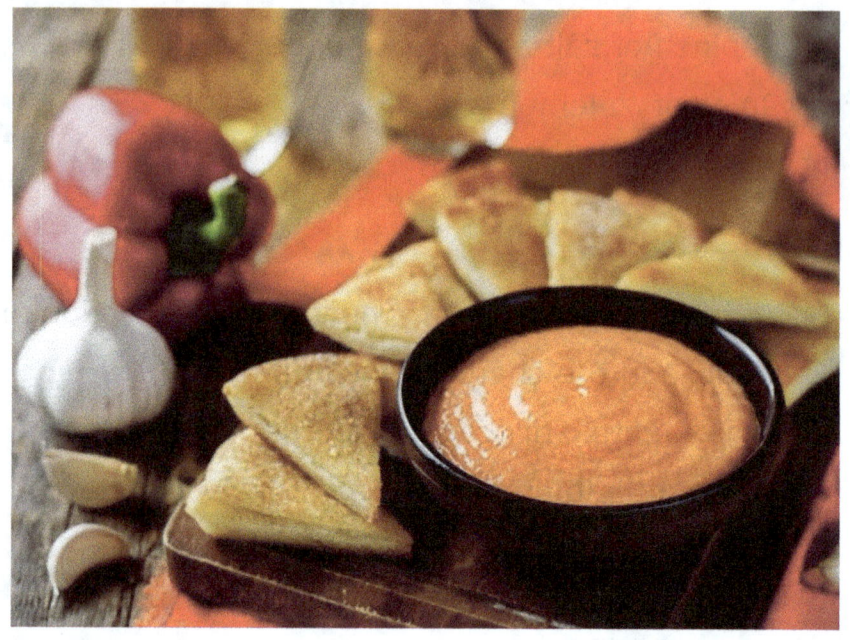

Preparation time: 10 minutes

Cooking time: 10 minutes

Servings: 4

Ingredients:

- ½ cup cashew cheese, grated
- 7 ounces roasted red peppers, chopped
- 2 tablespoons parsley, chopped

- 2 tablespoons olive oil
- ¼ cup capers, drained
- 1 tablespoon lemon juice

Directions:

1. Heat up a pan with the oil over medium heat, add the peppers and the other ingredients, stir, cook for 10 minutes and take off the heat.
2. Blend using an immersion blender, divide the mix into bowls and serve.

Nutrition:

calories 95, fat 8.6, fiber 1.2, carbs 4.7, protein 1.4

Cherry shed Coconut Muffins

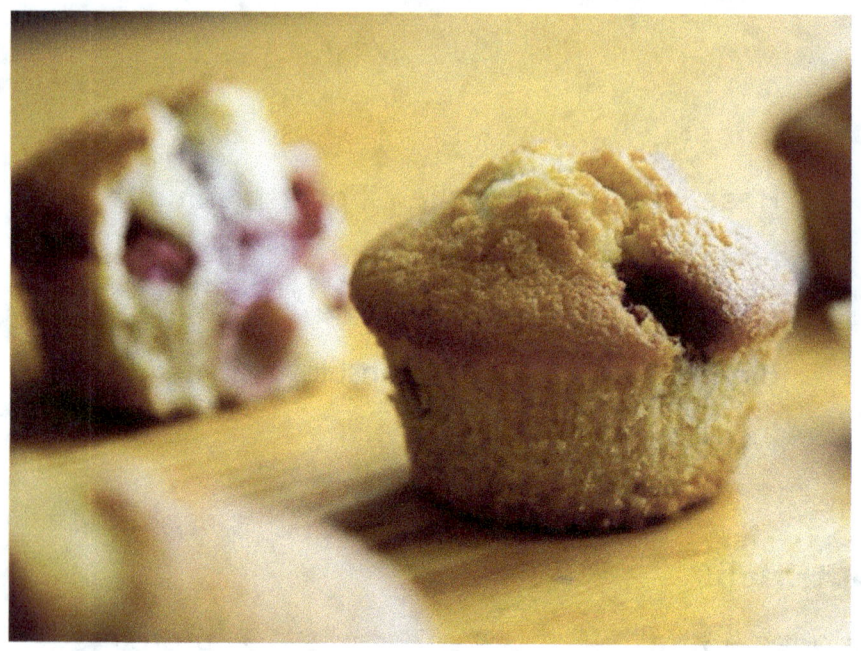

Preparation Time: 15 minutes

Cooking Time: 30 minutes

Servings: 12

Ingredients:

- ½ c. coconut oil
- ½ mashed avocado
- 1 c. coconut sugar

- 1 tsp. almond extract
- 1 c. toasted almonds
- 2 c. coconut flour
- 2 tsps. Baking powder
- ½ tsp. salt
- 2 c. chopped cherries

Directions:

1. Preheat oven to 375 °F. In a bowl, beat coconut butter and Stevia (or coconut sugar). Add a smashed avocado and mix well.
2. In a separate bowl, combine together dry ingredients and add them to the mixture.
3. Stir in almond extract, almonds and cherries.
4. Pour muffin batter into 12 greased muffin cups.
5. Bake muffins for 30 minutes.
6. Serve warm or cold.

Nutrition:

Calories: 7, Fat: 14.82g, Carbs: 5.79g, Protein: 2.89g

Zaatar Popcorn

Preparation Time: 10 minutes

Cooking Time: 0 minute

Servings: 8

Ingredients:

- 8 cups popped popcorns
- 1/4 cup za'atar spice blend
- ¾ teaspoon salt
- 4 tablespoons olive oil

Directions:

1. Place all the ingredients except for popcorns in a large bowl and whisk until combined.
2. Then add popcorns, toss until well coated, and serve straight away.

Nutrition:

Calories:150 Cal, Fat: 9 g, Carbs: 15 g, Protein: 2 g, Fiber: 4 g

Rice Pizza

Preparation Time: 10 minutes

Cooking Time: 35 minutes

Servings: 6

Ingredients:

For the crust:

- 1 1/2 cup short-grain rice, cooked
- 1/2 teaspoon garlic powder
- 1 tablespoon red chili flakes
- 1 teaspoon coconut sugar

For the sauce:

- 1/4 teaspoon onion powder
- 1 tablespoon nutritional yeast
- 1/4 teaspoon ginger powder
- 1/4 teaspoon garlic powder
- 1 tablespoon red chili flakes
- 1 teaspoon soy sauce
- 1/2 cup tomato purée

For the toppings:

- 2 1/2 cups oyster mushrooms
- 2 scallions, sliced

- 1 chili pepper, deseeded, sliced
- 1 teaspoon coconut sugar
- 1 teaspoon soy sauce
- Baby corn as needed

Directions:

1. Prepare the crust and for this, place all of its ingredients in a bowl and stir until well combined.
2. Then take a pizza pan, line it with a parchment sheet, place rice mixture in it, spread it evenly, and then bake for 20 minutes at 350 degrees F.
3. Then spread tomato sauce over the crust, top evenly with remaining ingredients for the topping and continue baking for 15 minutes.
4. When done, slice the pizza into wedges and serve.

Nutrition:

Calories: 1 Cal, Fat: 5 g, Carbs: 30 g, Protein: 3 g, Fiber: 1 g

Chaffles With Keto Ice Cream

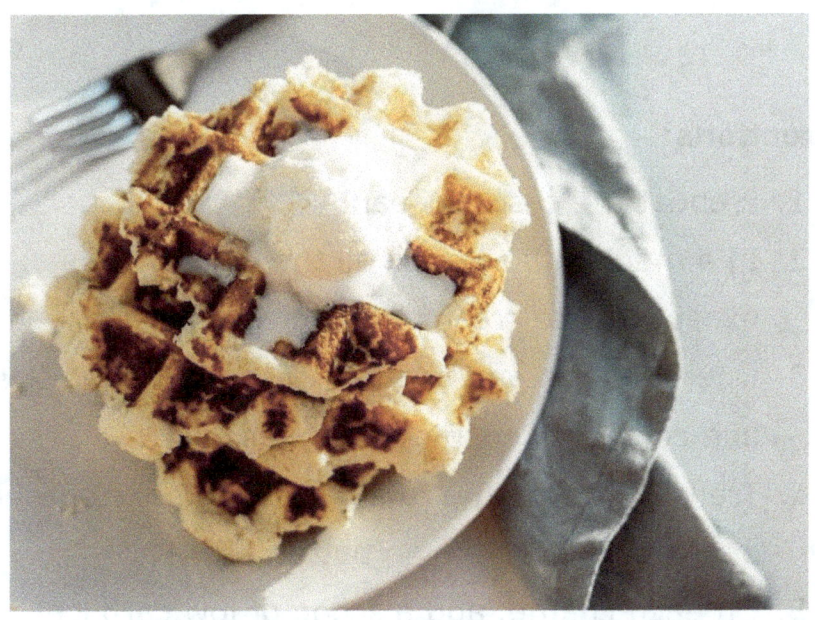

Preparation Time: 10 minutes

Cooking Time: 14 minutes

Servings: 2

Ingredients:

- 1 egg, beaten
- ¼ cup almond flour
- ½ cup finely grated mozzarella cheese
- 2 tbsp swerve confectioner's sugar

- 1/8 tsp xanthan gum
- Low-carb ice cream (flavor of your choice) for serving

Directions:

1. Preheat the cast iron pan.
2. In a medium bowl, mix all the ingredients except the ice cream.
3. Open the iron and add half of the mixture. Close and cook until crispy, 7 minutes.
4. Transfer the chaffle to a plate and make second one with the remaining batter.
5. On each chaffle, add a scoop of low carb ice cream, fold into half-moons and enjoy.

Nutrition:

Calories 89, Fats 6.48g, Carbs 1.67g, Net Carbs 1.37g, Protein 5.91g

Cauliflower Rice

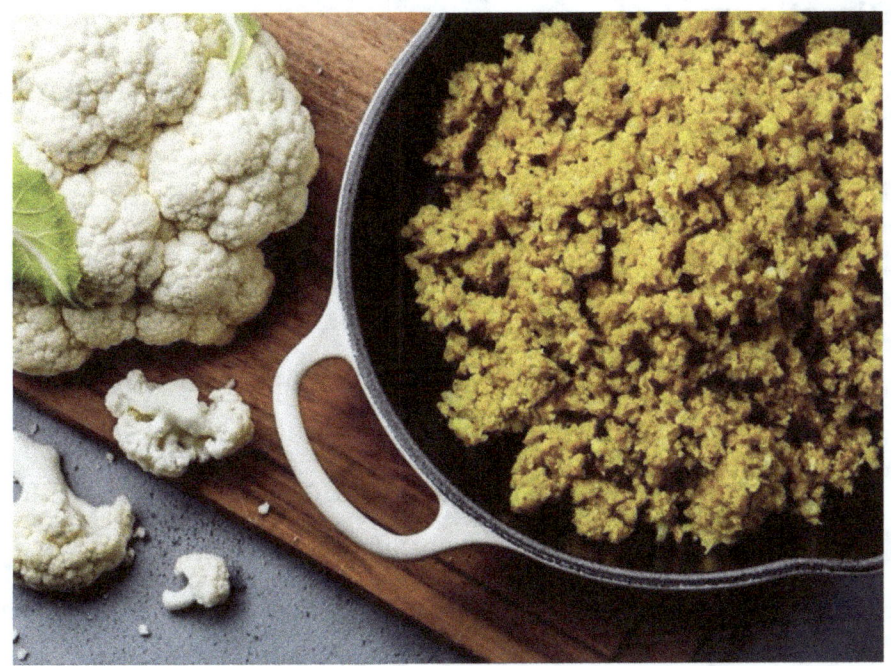

Preparation time: 15 minutes

Cooking time: 10 minutes

Servings: 2

Ingredients:

- ½ head cauliflower
- 1 tablespoon grass-fed butter
- ⅛ teaspoon freshly ground black pepper

- ½ teaspoon salt

Directions:

1. Wash the cauliflower under cold water. Pat dry with paper towels.
2. Chop the cauliflower into 1-inch pieces and put in a food processor. Pulse until the size of small rice.
3. Place a small griddle over medium-high heat. Melt the butter and add the cauliflower. Season with the salt and pepper and cook for 7 to 8 minutes, or until the cauliflower is tender.

Nutrition:

calories 74, fat 6g, protein 1g, carbs 4g, fiber 2g, sugar 2g, sodium 642mg

Queso Blanco Dip

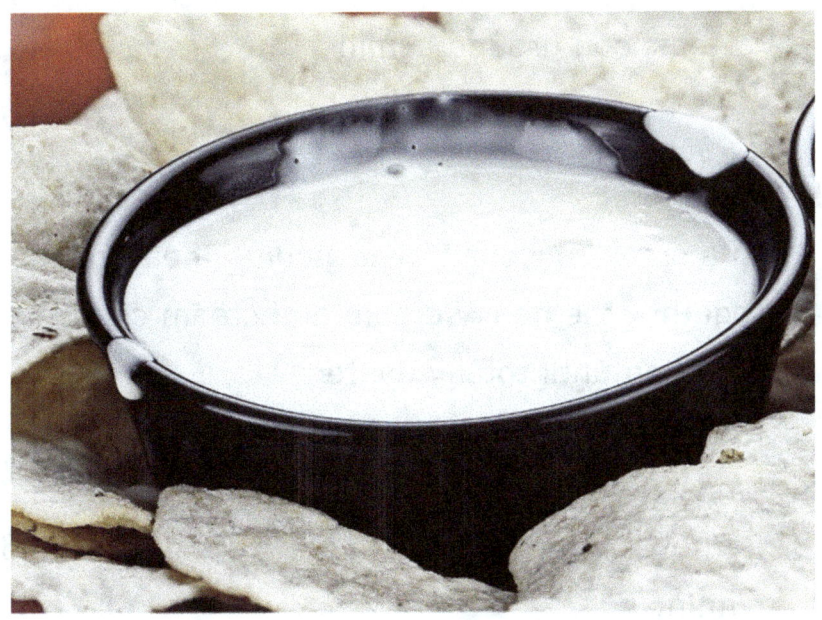

Preparation time: 5 minutes

Cooking time: 10 minutes

Servings: 8

Ingredients:

- ½ cup heavy (whipping) cream
- 1 cup shredded Monterey Jack cheese
- 3 ounces cream cheese
- 1 cup shredded queso blanco or other sharp

white cheddar cheese
- 1 (4.5-ounce) can diced green chiles, drained
- ½ teaspoon freshly ground black pepper
- ½ teaspoon ground cumin

Directions:
1. In a small saucepan over medium heat, melt together the heavy cream and cream cheese, whisking until totally melted.
2. Stir in the Monterey Jack cheese and queso blanco and the green chiles.
3. Remove from the heat and add the pepper and cumin.
4. Stir well and serve.

Nitritions:

calories 202, fat 18g, protein 8g, carbs 2g, fiber 0g, sugar 1g, sodium 265mg

Classic Buttermilk Syrup

Preparation time: 5 minutes

Cooking time: 10 minutes

Servings: 12

Ingredients:
- ¾ cup grass-fed butter
- ½ cup heavy (whipping) cream
- ¾ teaspoon white distilled vinegar
- 1 cup powdered monk fruit
- ¼ cup water
- ⅛ teaspoon salt
- 1 teaspoon baking soda
- 1 teaspoon vanilla extract

Directions:
1. In a large saucepan over medium heat, melt the butter.
2. In a small bowl, mix together the heavy cream and vinegar. Allow to sit for 5 minutes.
3. Add the water and monk fruit to the butter, whisking until all the sweetener has dissolved.

4. Add the cream mixture and salt to the pan, continuing to whisk while bringing the mixture to a gentle boil.
5. Remove the pan from the heat and stir in the baking soda and vanilla. Keep an eye on it because it will foam up. Whisk until all the foam is gone.
6. Serve warm.

Nutrition:

calories 137, fat 15g, protein 0g, carbs 0g, fiber 0g, sugar 0g, sodium 133mg, erythritol carbs 16g

Cheese Fries

Preparation Time: 5 minutes

Cooking Time: 4 minutes

Servings: 4

Ingredients:

- 8-ounces halloumi cheese, sliced into fries
- 1 serving marinara sauce, low carb
- 2-ounces tallow

Directions:

1. Heat the tallow in a pan over medium heat. Gently place halloumi pieces in the pan.
2. Cook halloumi fries for 2 minutes on each side or until lightly golden brown.
3. Serve with marinara sauce and enjoy!

Nutrition:

Calories: 200 Sugar: 0.3 g Fat: 18 g Carbohydrates: 1 g Cholesterol: 42 mg Protein: 12 g

Lemon Garlic Mushrooms

Preparation Time: 10 minutes

Cooking Time: 15 minutes

Servings: 4

Ingredients:

- 3 oz enoki mushrooms
- 6 oyster mushrooms, halved
- 5 oz cremini mushrooms, sliced
- 1 tbsp olive oil
- 1 tsp lemon zest, chopped
- 2 tbsp lemon juice
- 3 garlic cloves, sliced
- 1/2 red chili, sliced
- 1/2 onion, sliced
- 1 tsp sea salt

Directions:

1. Heat olive oil in a pan over high heat.
2. Add shallots, enoki mushrooms, oyster mushrooms, cremini mushrooms, and chili.

3. Stir well and cook over medium-high heat for 10 minutes.
4. Add lemon zest and stir well.
5. Season with lemon juice and salt and cook for 3-4 minutes.
6. Serve and enjoy.

Nutrition:

Calories 87 Fat 5.6 g Carbohydrates 7.5 g Sugar 1.8 g Protein 3 g Cholesterol 8 mg

Cauliflower Asparagus Soup

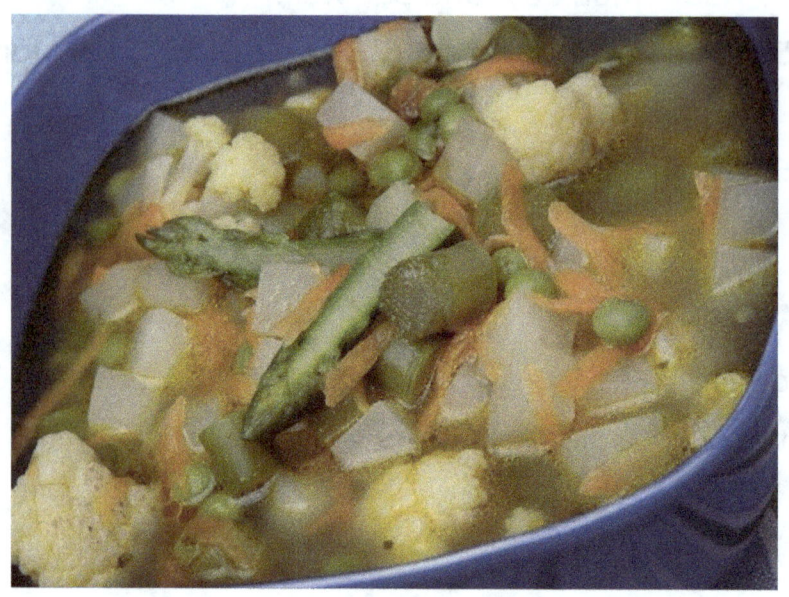

Preparation Time: 10 minutes

Cooking Time: 20 minutes

Servings: 4

Ingredients:

- 20 asparagus spears, chopped
- ½ cauliflower head, chopped
- 4 cups vegetable stock
- 2 garlic cloves, chopped

- 1 tbsp coconut oil
- Pepper
- Salt

Directions:

1. Heat coconut oil in a large saucepan over medium heat.
2. Add garlic and sauté until softened.
3. Add cauliflower, vegetable stock, pepper, and salt. Stir well and bring to boil.
4. Reduce heat to low and simmer for 20 minutes.
5. Add chopped asparagus and cook until softened.
6. Puree the soup using an immersion blender until smooth and creamy.
7. Stir well and serve warm.

Nutrition:

Calories 74 Fat 5.6 g Carbohydrates 8.9 g Sugar 5.1 g Protein 3.4 g Cholesterol 2 mg

Chard And Sweet Potato Soup

Preparation time: 10 minutes

Cooking time: 8 hours

Servings: 6

Ingredients:

- 1 yellow onion, chopped
- 1 tablespoon olive oil
- 1 carrot, chopped
- 2 garlic cloves, minced
- 4 sweet potatoes, cubed
- 1 celery stalk, chopped
- 1 bunch Swiss chard, leaves torn
- 1 cup brown lentils, dried
- 6 cups veggie stock
- 1 tablespoon coconut aminos
- Salt and black pepper to the taste

Directions:

1. In your slow cooker, mix oil with onion, carrot, celery, chard, garlic, potatoes, lentils, stock, salt, pepper and aminos, stir, cover and cook on

Low for 8 hours.
2. Ladle soup into bowls and serve right away.
3. Enjoy!
4. Salt and black pepper to the taste

Nutrition:

calories 312, fat 5, fiber 7, carbs 10, protein 5

Lentils Curry

Preparation time: 10 minutes

Cooking time: 6 hours

Servings: 8

Ingredients:
- 10 ounces spinach
- 2 cups red lentils
- 15 ounces canned tomatoes, chopped
- 1 tablespoon garlic, minced
- 2 cups cauliflower florets
- 1 teaspoon ginger, grated
- 1 yellow onion, chopped
- 4 cups veggie stock
- 2 tablespoons curry paste
- ½ teaspoon coriander, ground
- ½ teaspoon cumin, ground
- 2 teaspoons stevia
- A pinch of salt and black pepper
- ¼ cup cilantro, chopped
- 1 tablespoon lime juice

Directions:

1. In your slow cooker, mix spinach with lentils, garlic, tomatoes, cauliflower, ginger, onion, stock, curry paste, cumin, coriander, stevia, salt, pepper and lime juice, stir, cover and cook on Low for 6 hours.
2. Add cilantro, stir, divide into bowls and serve.
3. Enjoy!

Nutrition:

calories 105, fat 1, fiber 7, carbs 22, protein 7

Flax Egg (vegan)

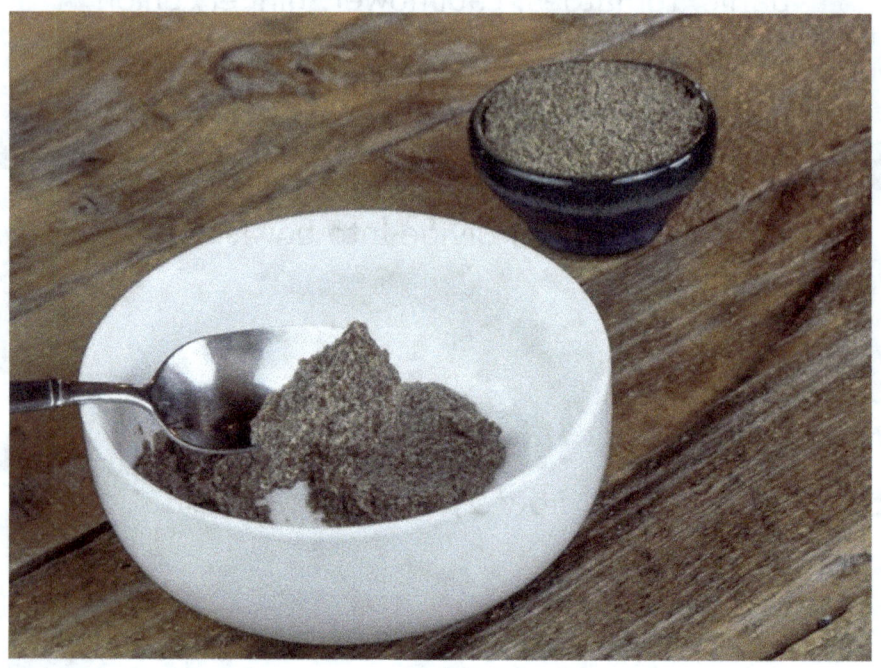

Preparation Time: 12 minutes

Cooking Time: 0 minute

Servings: 1

Ingredients:
- 1 tbsp. ground flaxseed
- 2-3 tbsp. lukewarm water

Directions:

1. Mix the ground flaxseed and water in a small bowl by using a spoon.
2. Cover the mixture and let it sit for 10 minutes.
3. Use the flax egg immediately, or, store it in an airtight container in the fridge and consume within 5 days.

Nutrition:

Calories: 37kcal, Net Carbs: 0.2g, Fat: 2.7g, Protein: 1.1g, Fiber: 1.9g, Sugar: 0g

Maple-Walnut Oatmeal Cookies

Preparation time: 5 minutes

cooking time: 10 minutes

servings: about 2 dozen cookies

Ingredients

- 1 1/2 cups whole-grain flour
- 1 teaspoon baking powder
- 1/4 teaspoon ground nutmeg
- 1 1/2 cups old-fashioned oats
- 1/8 teaspoon salt
- 1 teaspoon ground cinnamon
- 1 cup chopped walnuts
- 1/2 cup vegan margarine, melted
- 1/2 cup pure maple syrup
- 1/4 cup light brown sugar
- 2 teaspoons pure vanilla extract

Directions

1. Preheat the oven to 375 °F. In a large bowl, sift together the flour, baking powder, salt, cinnamon, and nutmeg. Stir in the oats and

walnuts.
2. In a medium bowl, combine the margarine, maple syrup, sugar, and vanilla and mix well.
3. Add the wet Ingredients to the dry Ingredients, stirring to mix well.
4. Drop the cookie dough by the tablespoonful onto an ungreased baking sheet and press down slightly with a fork.
5. Bake until browned, 10 to 12 minutes.
6. Cool the cookies slightly before transferring to a wire rack to cool completely.
7. Store in an airtight container.

Cherry-Vanilla Rice Pudding (Pressure cooker

Preparation time: 5 minutes

Servings: 4-6

Ingredients

- 1 cup short-grain brown rice
- 1¾ cups nondairy milk, plus more as needed
- 1½ cups water
- 1 teaspoon vanilla extract (use ½ teaspoon if you use vanilla milk
- 4 tablespoons unrefined sugar or pure maple syrup (use 2 tablespoons if you use a sweetened milk), plus more as needed
- Pinch salt
- ¼ cup dried cherries or ½ cup fresh or frozen pitted cherries

Directions

1. In your electric pressure cooker's cooking pot, combine the rice, milk, water, sugar, vanilla, and salt.

2. High pressure for 30 minutes. Close and lock the lid and ensure the pressure valve is sealed, then select High Pressure and set the time for 30 minutes.
3. Pressure Release. Once the cook time is complete, let the pressure release naturally, about 20 minutes. Once all the pressure has released, carefully unlock and remove the lid. Stir in the cherries and put the lid back on loosely for about 10 minutes.
4. Serve, adding more milk or sugar, as desired.

Nutrition

Calories: 177; Total fat: 1g; Protein: 3g; Sodium: 27mg; Fiber: 2g

Strawberry Parfaits With Cashew Crème

Preparation time: 10 minutes • chill time: 50 minutes •

servings: 4

Ingredients

- 1/2 cup unsalted raw cashews
- 4 tablespoons light brown sugar
- 1/2 cup plain or vanilla soy milk
- ¾ cup firm silken tofu, drained
- 2 cups sliced strawberries
- 1 teaspoon pure vanilla extract
- 1 teaspoon fresh lemon juice
- Fresh mint leaves, for garnish

Directions

1. In a blender, grind the cashews and 3 tablespoons of the sugar to a fine powder. Add the soy milk and blend until smooth. Add the tofu and vanilla and continue to blend until smooth and creamy.

2. Scrape the cashew mixture into a medium bowl, cover, and refrigerate for 30 minutes.
3. In a large bowl, combine the strawberries, lemon juice, and remaining 1 tablespoon sugar. Stir gently to combine and set aside at room temperature for 20 minutes.
4. Spoon alternating layers of the strawberries and cashew crème into parfait glasses or wine glasses, ending with a dollop of the cashew crème.
5. Garnish with mint leaves and serve.

Vegan Chocolate Bars

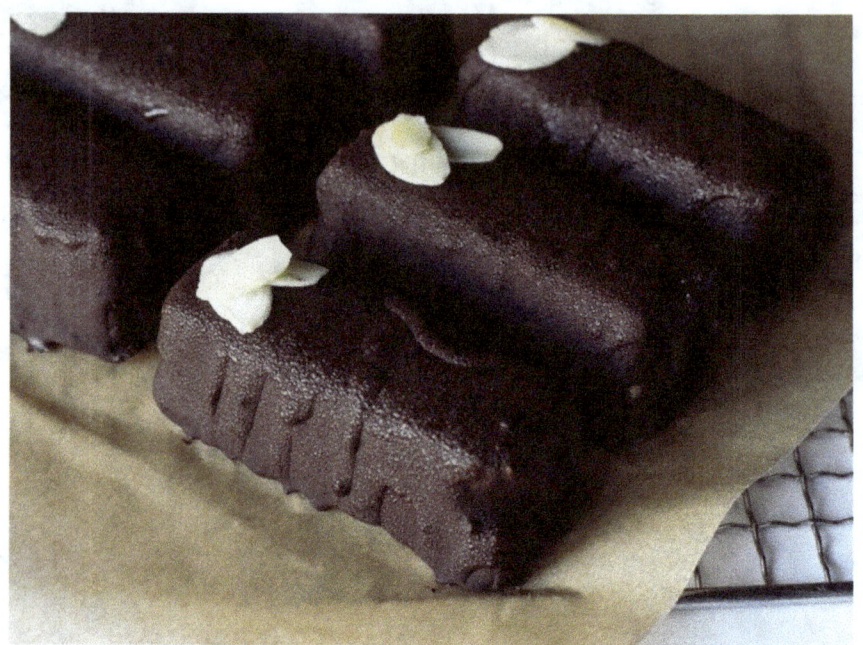

Preparation time: 10 minutes

Cooking Time: 1 hour

Servings: 3

Ingredients:

- 2 lbs. summer squash, cut into 1-inch pieces
- 1/8 tsp garlic powder
- 1/8 tsp pepper

- 3 tbsp olive oil
- 1 large lemon juice
- 1/8 tsp paprika
- Pepper
- Salt

Directions:

1. Preheat the oven to 400 F/ 204 C.
2. Spray a baking tray with cooking spray.
3. Place squash pieces onto the prepared baking tray and drizzle with olive oil.
4. Season with paprika, pepper, and garlic powder.
5. Squeeze lemon juice over the squash and bake in preheated oven for 50-60 minutes.
6. Serve hot and enjoy.

Nutrition:

Calories 182 Fat 15 g Carbohydrates 12.3 g Sugar 11 g Protein 3.2 g Cholesterol 0 mg;

Pina-Colada Cake.

Preparation Time: 20 Minutes

Servings: 6

Ingredients:

- 2 cups unbleached all-purpose flour
- 1 cup cream of coconut
- 1 cup confectioners' sugar
- ¾ cup canned pineapple, well drained, juice reserved
- ⅓ cup packed light brown sugar or granulated natural sugar
- ¼ cup unsweetened shredded coconut
- 1 tablespoon dark rum or 1 teaspoon rum extract
- 3 tablespoons vegan butter, softened, or vegetable oil
- 1½ teaspoons baking powder
- 1 teaspoon apple cider vinegar
- ½ teaspoon salt
- ½ teaspoon baking soda
- ½ teaspoon coconut extract

Directions:

1. Lightly oil a baking tray that will fit in the steamer basket of your Cooker.
2. In a bowl combine the flour, sugar, shredded coconut, baking soda, baking powder, and salt.
3. In another bowl, combine the cream of coconut, pineapple juice and flesh, rum, vinegar, and coconut extract.
4. Combine the wet and dry mixes and stir well to ensure they are evenly combined.
5. Pour the batter into your baking tray and put the tray in your steamer basket.
6. Pour the minimum amount of water into the base of your Cooker and lower the steamer basket.
7. Seal and cook on Steam for 12 minutes.
8. Release the pressure quickly and set to one side to cool a little.
9. When the cake is cool glaze with a light mix of confectioners' sugar and water.

Chocolate Almond Butter Smoothie

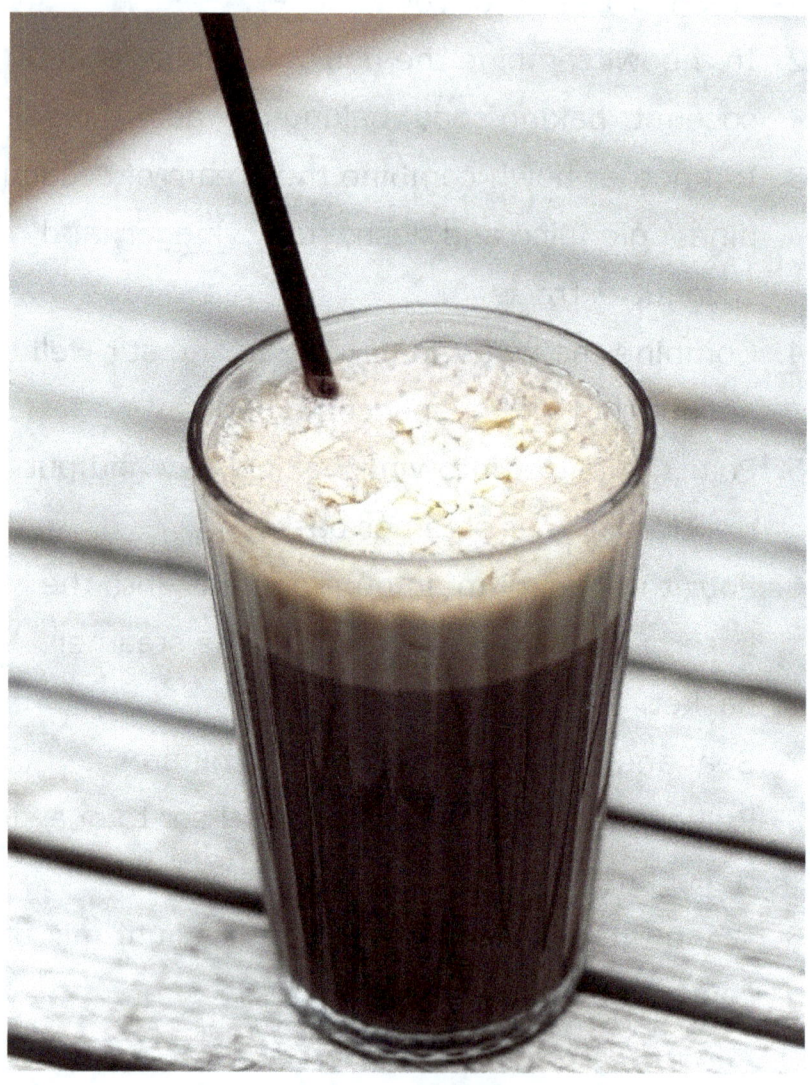

Preparation time: 35 minutes

Ingredients:

- 2 tbsp. chocolate protein powder
- ½ tbsp. cacao powder
- 2 tbsp. almond butter
- 1 cup almond milk
- 1 fresh banana
- ½ cup fresh strawberries
- 1 tbsp. chia or hemp seeds
- Maple syrup or stevia for sweetening

Directions:

1. Put all the ingredients into the blender and mix until it has creamy consistency.

Nutmeg Pudding

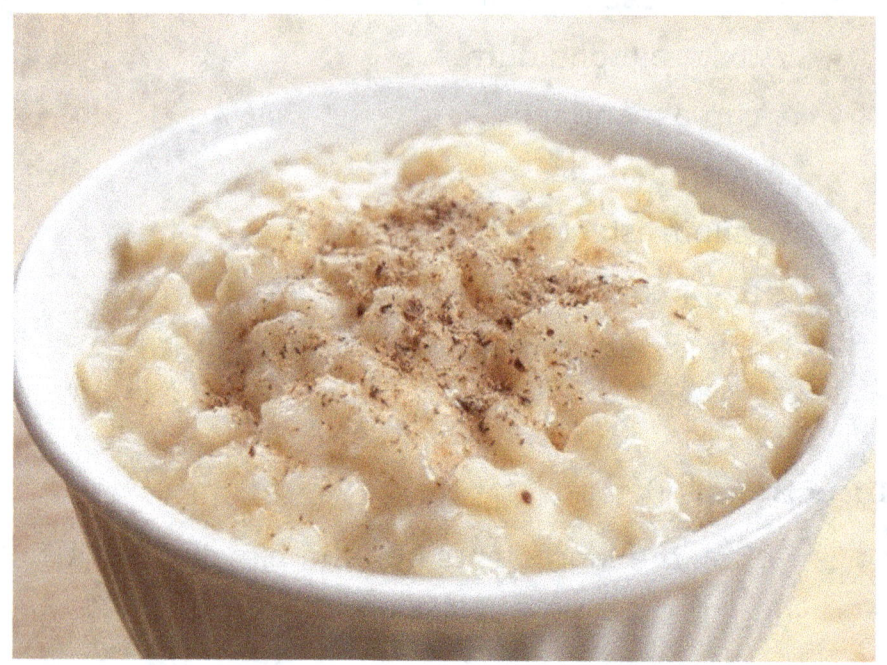

Preparation time: 10 minutes

Cooking time: 20 minutes

Servings: 6

Ingredients:

- 1 cup cauliflower rice
- 2 tablespoons stevia
- 1 teaspoon nutmeg, ground

- 2 tablespoons flaxseed mixed with 3 tablespoons water
- 2 cups almond milk
- ¼ teaspoon nutmeg, grated

Directions:

1. In a pan, combine the cauliflower rice with the flaxseed mix and the other ingredients, whisk, cook over medium heat for 20 minutes, divide into bowls and serve cold.

Nutrition:

calories 220, fat 6.6, fiber 3.4, carbs 12.4, protein 3.4

Grapes Vanilla Cream

Preparation time: 1 hour

Cooking time: 0 minutes

Servings: 4

Ingredients:

- 1 cup coconut cream
- 2 cups almond milk
- 1 cup grapes, halved
- 3 tablespoons stevia
- 1 teaspoon vanilla extract
- 1 teaspoon gelatin powder

Directions:

1. In a bowl, combine the grapes with the coconut cream, the almond milk and the other ingredients, whisk well, divide into cups and keep in the fridge for 1 hour before serving.

Nutrition:

calories 432, fat 43, fiber 4.2, carbs 14, protein 4.3

Chocolate Fudge

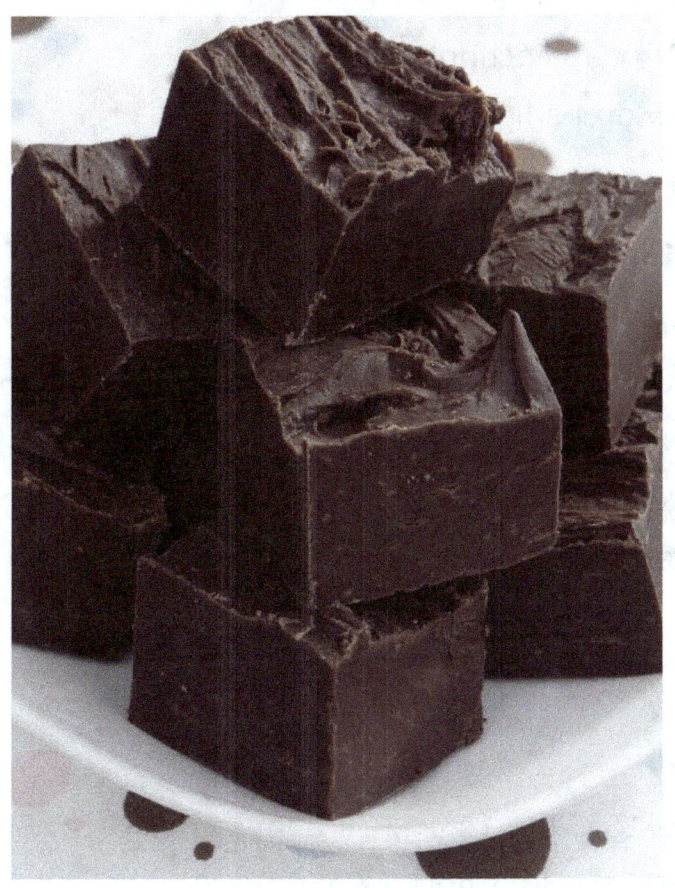

Preparation Time: 10 minutes

Cooking Time: 0 minute

Servings: 12

Ingredients:

- 4 oz unsweetened dark chocolate
- 1 tsp vanilla extract
- 3/4 cup coconut butter
- 15 drops liquid stevia

Directions:

1. Melt coconut butter and dark chocolate.
2. Add ingredients to the large bowl and combine well.
3. Pour mixture into a silicone loaf pan and place in refrigerator until set.
4. Cut into pieces and serve.

Nutrition:

Calories 157, Fat 14.1g, Carbohydrates 6.1g, Sugar 1g, Protein 2.3g, Cholesterol 0mg

NOTE

www.ingramcontent.com/pod-product-compliance
Lightning Source LLC
Chambersburg PA
CBHW070102120526
44589CB00033B/1483